Egg Quality Diet Book

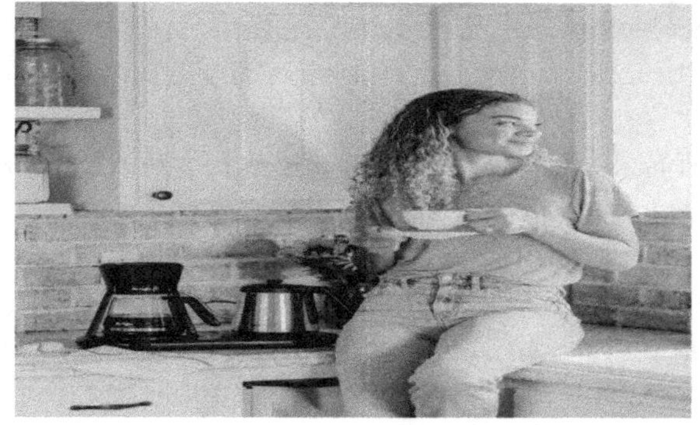

Natural Ways to Boost Fertility and
Get Pregnant Recipes & Meal Plan

Troy Clay

Table of Contents

INTRODUCTION

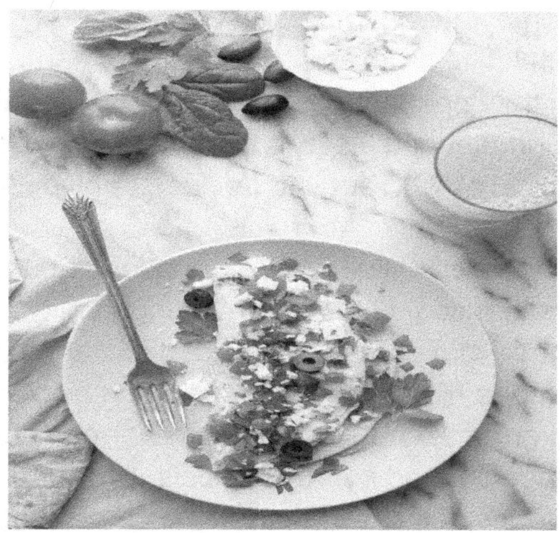

As a young woman, Julianne had always taken her health for granted. She ate whatever she wanted, skipped meals when she was busy, and never gave a second thought to the quality of the food she consumed. That all changed when she decided to start trying for a baby.

At her first prenatal appointment, Julianne was surprised to learn that her egg quality was lower than it should be. Her doctor explained that this could make it more difficult for her to conceive and increase the risk of miscarriage. Julianne was determined to do everything in her power to improve her egg quality and increase her chances of having a healthy baby.

That's when she stumbled upon a groundbreaking new book called "Egg Quality Diet." This book, written by a team of fertility experts and nutritionists, promised to provide women with the tools they needed to improve their egg quality through diet and lifestyle changes. Julianne was sceptical at first, but she decided to give it a try.

The book was filled with information about the foods that could help improve egg quality, as well as those that should be avoided. Julianne learned that foods high in antioxidants, such as berries and leafy greens, could help protect her eggs from damage caused by free radicals. She also learned that foods rich in healthy fats, such as avocado and nuts, could help support the production of hormones that were essential for ovulation.

But the book wasn't just about what to eat - it also provided tips on how to live a healthier lifestyle. Julianne learned the importance of getting enough sleep, managing stress through meditation and yoga, and avoiding environmental toxins that could negatively impact her fertility.

As Julianne began implementing the recommendations in the book, she noticed a significant improvement in her overall health and wellbeing. She had more energy throughout the day, slept better at night, and felt more focused and productive at work. But most importantly, she saw improvements in her egg quality as well. Her doctor confirmed that her eggs were now of higher quality, which increased her chances of conceiving and carrying a healthy baby to term.

Julianne's experience inspired her to share the knowledge she had gained with other women who were struggling with fertility issues. She started a blog where she shared recipes, tips, and resources related to fertility nutrition and lifestyle changes. Her blog quickly gained a following, and Julianne became known as an expert in the field of fertility nutrition.

Years later, Julianne gave birth to a healthy baby girl - a testament to the power of diet and lifestyle changes in improving fertility outcomes. She continued to spread the word about the importance of egg quality diet and lifestyle changes through her blog and social media channels, helping countless other women on their own fertility journeys.

Explanation of the importance of egg Quality Diet for Fertility

Egg quality is a crucial factor in determining the success rate of fertility treatments such as in vitro fertilisation (IVF) and intracytoplasmic sperm injection (ICSI). The quality of the eggs produced by a woman's ovaries is a significant determinant of her chances of conceiving naturally or through assisted reproductive technologies. Therefore, it is essential to maintain a diet rich in nutrients that promote egg quality for women trying to conceive.

The process of ovulation involves the maturation of an egg in the ovary, which takes approximately 120 days. During this time, the follicle containing the egg undergoes several changes, including cell division and the accumulation of nutrients. The nutrients required for these processes are obtained from the diet, and a deficiency in any of these nutrients can negatively impact egg quality.

Here are some essential nutrients that promote egg quality:

1. Folate: Folate, also known as vitamin B9, is essential for DNA synthesis and repair. Adequate folate intake before and during pregnancy reduces the risk of neural tube defects in the foetus. Studies have shown that women who consume high levels of folate have higher chances of conceiving and delivering a healthy baby.

2. Vitamin D: Vitamin D is necessary for calcium absorption and bone health. Recent studies have shown that vitamin D may also improve egg quality by increasing the levels of progesterone, a hormone that supports embryo implantation.

3. Omega-3 fatty acids: Omega-3 fatty acids are essential fats that are important for brain development and cardiovascular health. Studies have shown that omega-3 fatty acids may improve egg quality by reducing inflammation and oxidative stress, which can damage the eggs.

4. Antioxidants: Antioxidants such as vitamin C, vitamin E, and beta-carotene help protect the body from oxidative stress, which can damage cells and DNA. Oxidative stress can negatively impact egg quality, leading to decreased fertility. Therefore, consuming foods rich in antioxidants can help improve egg quality and increase fertility.

5. Protein: Protein is essential for tissue growth and repair, including the development of follicles and eggs. Women trying to conceive should aim to consume high-quality protein sources such as lean meats, poultry, beans, and lentils to support egg quality and overall reproductive health.

In conclusion, maintaining a diet rich in folate, vitamin D, omega-3 fatty acids, antioxidants, and protein is crucial for promoting egg quality and improving fertility. Women trying to conceive should aim to consume a balanced diet that includes a variety of whole foods to support overall reproductive health. Consulting with a healthcare provider or registered dietitian can provide personalised recommendations based on individual needs and medical history.

Brief overview of the book's content and structure

The Egg Quality Diet Book is a comprehensive guide that focuses on improving the quality of eggs in women who are trying to conceive. The book is written by Troy Clay, a renowned fertility expert and acupuncturist, and her team of nutritionists and fertility specialists.

The book is divided into several sections, each addressing a specific aspect of egg quality and fertility. Here's a brief overview of the content and structure of the Egg Quality Diet Book:

1. Introduction: The book begins with an introduction that explains the importance of egg quality in fertility and how it can affect pregnancy outcomes. It also introduces the concept of the Egg Quality Diet, which aims to improve egg quality through dietary changes.

2. Understanding Egg Quality: This section provides an in-depth explanation of what egg quality is, how it is measured, and how it affects fertility. It also discusses the factors that can impact egg quality, such as age, lifestyle, and environmental toxins.

3. The Egg Quality Diet: This section outlines the key principles of the Egg Quality Diet, which includes eating foods rich in antioxidants, healthy fats, and protein, while avoiding foods that can harm egg quality, such as processed foods and alcohol. The section also provides meal plans and recipes to help readers implement the dietary changes.

4. Nutrients for Egg Quality: This section focuses on specific nutrients that are essential for egg quality, such as folate, vitamin D, omega-3 fatty acids, and CoQ10. It provides information on how these nutrients work in the body and how to ensure adequate intake through dietary sources or supplements.

5. Lifestyle Factors: This section discusses lifestyle factors that can impact egg quality, such as stress management, sleep hygiene, exercise, and environmental toxins. It provides practical tips on how to manage these factors to support optimal egg quality.

6. Supplements: This section addresses the role of supplements in supporting egg quality and fertility. It provides information on which supplements are recommended and which ones should be avoided during fertility treatments.

7. Conclusion: The book concludes with a summary of the key takeaways from each section and encourages readers to make sustainable dietary changes to support optimal egg quality and fertility outcomes.

Overall, the Egg Quality Diet Book is an informative and practical resource for women who are trying to conceive and want to improve their egg quality through dietary changes. Its evidence-based approach and practical advice make it a valuable resource for anyone looking to optimise their fertility health.

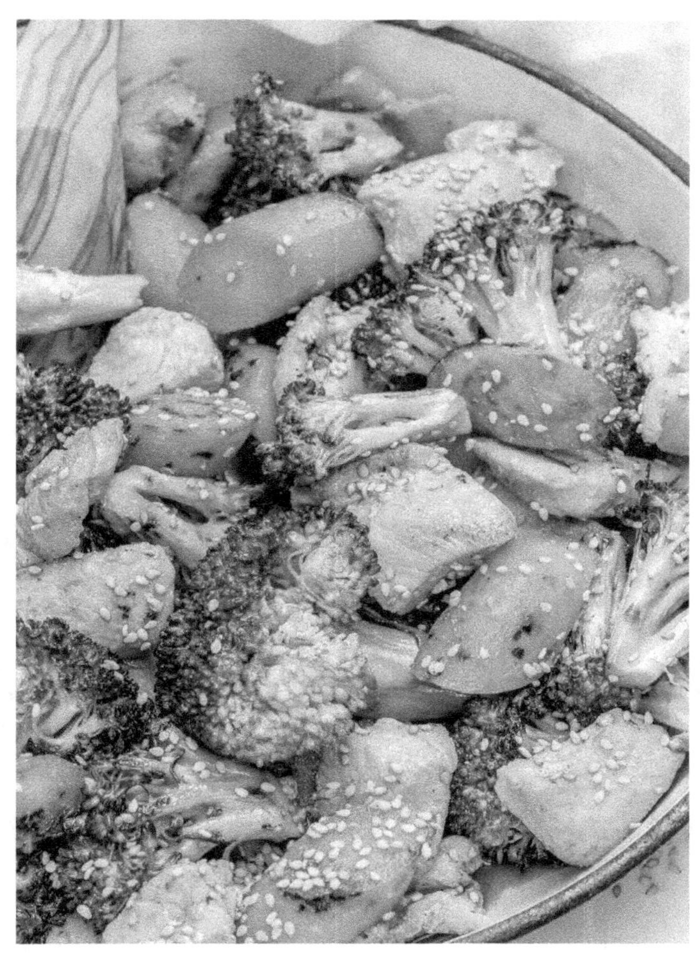

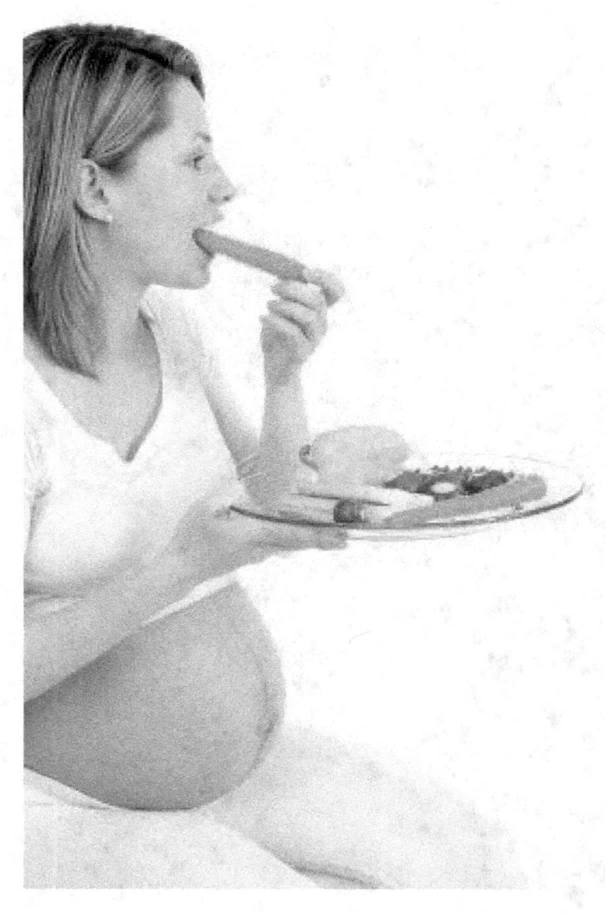

CHAPTER ONE

Understanding Egg Quality

Explanation of the factors that affect egg quality, including genetics, nutrition, and environment

Egg quality is a crucial factor that determines the fertilisation, development, and health of an embryo. The quality of an egg can be influenced by various factors, including genetics, nutrition, and environment. These aspects will be discussed in depth in this book.

Genetics

Genetics is the most significant factor that affects egg quality. Eggs are produced in the ovaries, and their quality is determined by the genetic makeup of the mother. Some women are born with a higher number of eggs that are of better quality, while others may have a lower number of poorer quality eggs. Genetic factors also play a role in determining the age at which a woman enters menopause, which can impact egg quality.

Nutrition

Nutrition is another crucial factor that affects egg quality. Adequate intake of essential nutrients is necessary for the production of high-quality eggs. Women who consume a healthy diet rich in vitamins, minerals, and antioxidants are more likely to produce healthy eggs. Some specific nutrients that are essential for egg quality include:

a) Folic acid: Folic acid is a B-vitamin that is essential for DNA synthesis and cell division. Adequate intake of folic acid before and during pregnancy can reduce the risk of birth defects and improve egg quality.

b) Vitamin D: Vitamin D is important for bone health and has been linked to improved egg quality. Women with low vitamin D levels may have a higher risk of infertility and poorer egg quality.

c) Omega-3 fatty acids: Omega-3 fatty acids are essential for brain health and have been linked to improved egg quality. Women who consume foods rich in omega-3 fatty acids, such as fatty fish and flaxseeds, may have higher-quality eggs.

d) Antioxidants: Antioxidants help protect cells from damage caused by free radicals. High levels of free radicals can lead to oxidative stress, which can negatively impact egg quality. Antioxidants such as vitamin C, vitamin E, and beta-carotene can help reduce oxidative stress and improve egg quality.

Environmental factors can also impact egg quality. Exposure to environmental toxins such as pesticides, pollution, and heavy metals can lead to oxidative stress and DNA damage in eggs, which can negatively impact fertility and pregnancy outcomes. Women who work in environments with high levels of environmental toxins may be at increased risk of poorer egg quality. Additionally, lifestyle factors such as smoking, alcohol consumption, and obesity can negatively impact egg quality.

In conclusion, several factors influence egg quality, including genetics, nutrition, and environment. Women who want to improve their chances of conceiving should focus on maintaining a healthy lifestyle that includes a nutritious diet rich in essential nutrients, avoiding environmental toxins where possible, and seeking medical advice if they have concerns about their fertility or egg quality. By taking these steps, women can increase their chances of producing high-quality eggs that will lead to a healthy pregnancy outcome.

The differences between high-quality and low-quality eggs

When it comes to fertility, the quality of eggs plays a crucial role in determining the success rate of in vitro fertilisation (IVF) treatments. While both high-quality and low-quality eggs can result in pregnancy, there are significant differences between the two that can impact fertility outcomes.

High-Quality Eggs

1. Maturity: High-quality eggs are fully mature, meaning they have completed meiosis and are ready for fertilisation. Mature eggs have a thicker zona pellucida (the outer layer of the egg) and a more compact cytoplasm (the jelly-like substance inside the egg).

2. Fewer Defects: Mature eggs are less likely to have defects such as abnormal chromosomes, which can lead to miscarriages or birth defects. High-quality eggs also have a lower risk of fragmentation, which occurs when the egg breaks into smaller pieces during the retrieval process.

3. Fertilisation Rate: Mature eggs are more likely to be successfully fertilised by sperm, resulting in higher fertilisation rates. This is because mature eggs have a better ability to bind with sperm and undergo the process of fertilisation.

4. Embryo Quality: High-quality eggs result in better embryo quality, which is essential for successful implantation and pregnancy. Embryos derived from high-quality eggs have a higher chance of developing into healthy embryos that can lead to successful implantation and pregnancy.

1. Immaturity: Low-quality eggs are immature, meaning they have not completed meiosis and are not ready for fertilisation. Immature eggs have a thinner zona pellucida and a more watery cytoplasm.

2. Higher Defects: Immature eggs are more likely to have defects such as abnormal chromosomes, which can lead to miscarriages or birth defects. Immature eggs also have a higher risk of fragmentation during the retrieval process.

3. Lower Fertilisation Rate: Immature eggs have a lower chance of being successfully fertilised by sperm due to their immaturity and lower ability to bind with sperm and undergo the process of fertilisation.

4. Lower Embryo Quality: Low-quality eggs result in lower embryo quality, which can negatively impact implantation and pregnancy outcomes. Embryos derived from low-quality eggs have a higher chance of developing into poor quality embryos that may not be able to successfully implant in the uterus or lead to pregnancy.

In conclusion, high-quality eggs are essential for successful IVF treatments due to their maturity, lower defects, higher fertilisation rates, and better embryo quality. While low-quality eggs can still result in pregnancy, they are associated with higher risks of chromosomal abnormalities, lower fertilisation rates, and lower embryo quality, which can negatively impact IVF outcomes. It is essential for patients undergoing IVF treatments to work closely with their healthcare providers to optimise their chances of success by focusing on producing high-quality eggs through various techniques such as ovarian stimulation, follicle monitoring, and egg maturation protocols.

CHAPTER TWO

The Role of Nutrition in Egg Quality

Explanation of the nutrients that are important for egg quality, including vitamins, minerals, and antioxidants

Egg quality is a crucial factor in achieving successful fertilisation and healthy embryo development. While genetics play a significant role in egg quality, dietary factors also contribute significantly. Adequate intake of certain vitamins, minerals, and antioxidants is essential for optimal egg quality. In this article, we will discuss the nutrients that are crucial for egg quality, including vitamins, minerals, and antioxidants.

- Vitamins

a) Vitamin D:
Vitamin D is essential for calcium absorption and bone health. It has also been found to improve egg quality by reducing the risk of miscarriage and promoting follicular development. Vitamin D deficiency has been linked to poor ovarian response and lower pregnancy rates in women undergoing IVF. Food sources of vitamin D include

fatty fish, fortified dairy products, and sunlight exposure.

b) Vitamin E:
Vitamin E is a powerful antioxidant that protects cells from oxidative stress. It has been found to improve egg quality by reducing oxidative damage to the eggs, which can impair fertilisation and embryo development. Food sources of vitamin E include nuts, seeds, and vegetable oils.

c) Vitamin C:
Vitamin C is another antioxidant that helps protect the eggs from oxidative stress. It also plays a role in collagen synthesis, which is essential for follicle growth and ovulation. Food sources of vitamin C include citrus fruits, berries, and leafy greens.

- Minerals

a) Zinc:
Zinc is an essential mineral for ovulation and follicular development. It helps regulate the menstrual cycle and promotes the production of oestrogen and progesterone. Zinc deficiency has been linked to poor ovarian response and lower pregnancy rates in women undergoing IVF. Zinc-rich foods include oysters, steak, and pumpkin seeds.

b) Magnesium:

Magnesium is a mineral that helps regulate the menstrual cycle and promote ovulation. It also plays a role in follicular development and reduces the risk of miscarriage. Magnesium deficiency has been linked to poor ovarian response and lower pregnancy rates in women undergoing IVF. Food sources of magnesium include leafy greens, nuts, and whole grains.

- Antioxidants

a) Coenzyme Q10 (CoQ10):
CoQ10 is a naturally occurring antioxidant that helps protect the eggs from oxidative stress. It also plays a role in mitochondrial function, which is essential for follicular development and ovulation. CoQ10 supplementation has been found to improve egg quality in women undergoing IVF. Food sources of CoQ10 include organ meats, fatty fish, and nuts.

b) Alpha-lipoic acid (ALA):
ALA is an antioxidant that helps protect the eggs from oxidative stress and improves insulin sensitivity, which can help regulate ovulation in women with polycystic ovary syndrome (PCOS). ALA supplementation has been found to improve egg quality in women undergoing IVF with PCOS. Food sources of ALA include broccoli, spinach, and potatoes.

In conclusion, adequate intake of vitamins D, E, C, minerals such as zinc and magnesium, and antioxidants such as CoQ10 and ALA are crucial for optimal egg quality. Incorporating these nutrients into a healthy diet can help improve fertility outcomes in women undergoing fertility treatments or trying to conceive naturally.

The foods and supplements that can improve egg quality

Egg quality is a crucial factor in achieving successful fertilisation and pregnancy. Poor egg quality can lead to difficulties in conceiving, miscarriages, and genetic abnormalities in the offspring. Fortunately, certain foods and supplements have been shown to improve egg quality, making them an essential part of a fertility-boosting diet.

1. Leafy Greens

Leafy greens such as spinach, kale, and broccoli are rich in folate, a B-vitamin that plays a crucial role in DNA synthesis and cell division. Folate deficiency has been linked to poor egg quality and an increased risk of chromosomal abnormalities. A study published in the Journal of Reproduction & Infertility found that women who consumed high levels of folate had better egg quality than those with lower intakes.

2. Berries

Berries such as strawberries, blueberries, and raspberries are rich in antioxidants called anthocyanins, which help protect the eggs from oxidative stress. Oxidative stress can damage the DNA in the eggs, leading to poor egg quality and infertility. A study published in the Journal of Agricultural and Food Chemistry found that consuming berries improved egg quality in mice by reducing oxidative stress levels.

3. Omega-3 Fatty Acids

Omega-3 fatty acids are essential fats that play a crucial role in brain development and heart health. They also have anti-inflammatory properties that can help reduce inflammation in the body, which is linked to poor egg quality. A study published in the Journal of Clinical Endocrinology & Metabolism found that women who consumed high levels of omega-3 fatty acids had better egg quality than those with lower intakes.

4. Coenzyme Q10 (CoQ10)

CoQ10 is a nutrient that is naturally produced by the body and plays a crucial role in energy production. It also has antioxidant properties that can help protect the eggs from oxidative stress. A study published in the Journal of Reproduction & Infertility found that women who supplemented with CoQ10 had better egg quality than those who did not.

5. Vitamin D

Vitamin D is a hormone that plays a crucial role in bone health and immune function. It also has anti-inflammatory properties that can help reduce inflammation in the body, which is linked to poor egg quality. A study published in the Journal of Clinical Endocrinology & Metabolism found that women who were supplemented with vitamin D had better egg quality than those who did not.

In conclusion, improving egg quality is essential for achieving successful fertilisation and pregnancy. Consuming foods rich in folate, berries, omega-3 fatty acids, CoQ10, and vitamin D can help improve egg quality by reducing oxidative stress, inflammation, and DNA damage. Incorporating these foods into a fertility-boosting diet can significantly improve the chances of conceiving and having a healthy baby.

CHAPTER THREE

Dietary Strategies for Improving Egg Quality

Specific dietary strategies that can improve egg quality, such as reducing oxidative stress, increasing omega-3 fatty acids, and improving insulin sensitivity

Egg quality is a crucial factor in fertility, as it directly affects the chances of successful conception and healthy embryo development. Several dietary strategies have been identified that can improve egg quality by reducing oxidative stress, increasing omega-3 fatty acids, and improving insulin sensitivity.

Reducing Oxidative Stress

Oxidative stress is a condition where the body produces excessive free radicals, which can damage cellular structures and impair reproductive function. High levels of oxidative stress have been linked to decreased egg quality and increased risk of miscarriage. To reduce oxidative stress, the following dietary strategies can be adopted:

1. Antioxidant-rich foods: Antioxidants such as vitamin C, vitamin E, and beta-carotene can help neutralise free radicals and prevent oxidative damage. Foods rich in antioxidants include berries, leafy greens, citrus fruits, nuts, and seeds.

2. Omega-3 fatty acids: Omega-3 fatty acids have been shown to have antioxidant properties and can help reduce oxidative stress. Fatty fish such as salmon, sardines, and mackerel, as well as flaxseeds, chia seeds, and walnuts, are high in omega-3 fatty acids.

3. Reduce exposure to environmental toxins: Environmental toxins such as pesticides, pollutants, and plastics can increase oxidative stress levels. Reducing exposure to these toxins by choosing organic produce, avoiding plastic containers, and using natural cleaning products can help reduce oxidative stress.

Increasing Omega-3 Fatty Acids

Omega-3 fatty acids are essential fats that play a crucial role in reproductive health. They have been shown to improve egg quality by reducing inflammation and oxidative stress levels. To increase omega-3 fatty acid intake, the following dietary strategies can be adopted:

1. Fatty fish: Omega-3 fatty acids are abundant in fatty fish such as salmon, sardines, and mackerel.

Consuming two servings of fatty fish per week can significantly increase omega-3 intake.

2. Flaxseeds: Flaxseeds are a rich source of alpha-linolenic acid (ALA), a type of omega-3 fatty acid. Adding ground flax seeds to oatmeal or yoghurt is an easy way to increase omega-3 intake.

3. Chia seeds: Chia seeds are another rich source of ALA. Adding chia seeds to smoothies or oatmeal is an easy way to increase omega-3 intake.

Improving Insulin Sensitivity

Insulin resistance is a condition where the body becomes less responsive to insulin, leading to high blood sugar levels. Insulin resistance has been linked to decreased egg quality and increased risk of miscarriage. To improve insulin sensitivity, the following dietary strategies can be adopted:

1. Low glycemic index foods: Foods with a low glycemic index (GI) release sugar into the bloodstream slowly, preventing spikes in blood sugar levels. Low GI foods include whole grains such as brown rice and quinoa, fruits such as berries and apples, and non-starchy vegetables such as broccoli and spinach.

2. Fibre: Fibre helps slow down the absorption of sugar into the bloodstream, preventing spikes in blood sugar levels. Consuming foods rich in fibre such as whole grains, fruits, and vegetables can help improve insulin sensitivity.

3. Regular exercise: Regular exercise helps improve insulin sensitivity by making the body more responsive to insulin. Aim for at least 150 minutes of moderate-intensity aerobic exercise per week or 75 minutes of vigorous-intensity aerobic exercise per week.

In conclusion, reducing oxidative stress, increasing omega-3 fatty acids intake, and improving insulin sensitivity through dietary strategies can significantly improve egg quality, leading to improved fertility outcomes for women undergoing fertility treatments or trying to conceive naturally.

Tips for implementing these strategies into a healthy diet

As women approach their late 30s and early 40s, they may start to worry about their fertility and the quality of their eggs. While genetics and age play a significant role in egg quality, dietary strategies can also make a difference. Here are some tips for implementing dietary strategies for improving egg quality:

- Eat a balanced diet A healthy and balanced diet is essential for overall health and wellbeing, including egg quality. Ensure

your diet includes a variety of whole foods,
such as fruits, vegetables, whole grains,
lean protein, and healthy fats.

- Including foods rich in antioxidants Antioxidants help protect the body from oxidative stress, which can damage eggs and lead to decreased fertility. Foods rich in antioxidants include berries, leafy greens, nuts, seeds, and dark chocolate.

- Limit processed foods Processed foods often contain added sugars, unhealthy fats, and preservatives that can negatively impact egg quality. Reduce your intake of processed foods and replace them with whole foods.

- Increased intake of omega-3 fatty acids Omega-3 fatty acids are essential for overall health and have been shown to improve egg quality. Good sources of omega-3s include fatty fish such as salmon, sardines, and mackerel, as well as flaxseeds and chia seeds.

- Limit caffeine intake Caffeine has been linked to decreased fertility and may also negatively impact egg quality. Limit your intake of caffeine to less than 200mg per day (about one 8-ounce cup of coffee).

- Stay hydrated, Dehydration can negatively impact fertility and may also impact egg quality. Drink plenty of water throughout the day to stay hydrated.

- Maintaining a healthy weight, Being overweight or underweight can negatively impact fertility and may also impact egg quality. Maintain a healthy weight by eating a well-balanced diet and exercising regularly.

- Avoid smoking and excessive alcohol consumption Smoking and excessive alcohol consumption can negatively impact fertility and may also impact egg quality. Avoid smoking and limit alcohol consumption to less than one drink per day (for women).

Incorporating these dietary strategies into your lifestyle can help improve egg quality and overall fertility health. Remember to always consult with a healthcare provider if you have concerns about your fertility or egg quality.

CHAPTER FOUR

The Impact of Lifestyle Factors on Egg Quality

Lifestyle factors that can affect egg quality, such as stress, alcohol consumption, and smoking

Egg quality is a crucial factor in fertility, as it determines the likelihood of successful implantation and pregnancy. While genetics play a significant role in egg quality, lifestyle factors can also have a significant impact. Here are some lifestyle factors that can affect egg quality:

1. Stress: Chronic stress can negatively impact egg quality by increasing levels of cortisol, a hormone that can disrupt the menstrual cycle and ovulation. High cortisol levels can also lead to the production of abnormal eggs, making it harder for them to fertilise and implant. To mitigate the effects of stress on egg quality, women can practise stress-reduction techniques such as meditation, yoga, or deep breathing exercises.

2. Alcohol consumption: Excessive alcohol consumption can impair egg quality by disrupting the reproductive cycle and reducing the number of mature eggs produced. Alcohol also interferes with the absorption of essential nutrients such as folate, which is crucial for healthy egg development. Women are advised to limit their alcohol intake to no more than one drink per day while trying to conceive.

3. Smoking: Smoking is known to decrease egg quality by reducing blood flow to the ovaries and increasing oxidative stress, which damages the DNA in eggs. Smoking also increases the risk of miscarriage and birth defects. Women who smoke are advised to quit smoking before trying to conceive to improve their chances of conceiving and having a healthy pregnancy.

4. Diet: A healthy diet rich in nutrients such as folate, vitamin D, and omega-3 fatty acids is essential for healthy egg development. Women should aim to consume a balanced diet with plenty of fruits, vegetables, whole grains, and lean protein sources. Supplements such as folic acid and prenatal vitamins can also help ensure adequate nutrient intake during the preconception period.

5. Exercise: Regular exercise is beneficial for overall health and can improve egg quality by promoting blood flow to the ovaries and reducing stress levels. However, excessive exercise or extreme dieting can lead to menstrual irregularities and disruptions in ovulation, which can negatively impact egg quality. Women are advised to maintain a healthy weight and engage in moderate exercise for optimal fertility health.

In conclusion, lifestyle factors such as stress, alcohol consumption, smoking, diet, and exercise can all affect egg quality. By making healthy lifestyle choices and managing stress levels, women can improve their chances of conceiving and having a healthy pregnancy. It's essential to consult with a healthcare provider for personalised advice on how lifestyle factors may impact fertility health based on individual circumstances.

Tips for managing Lifestyle factors to improve egg quality

Women's egg quality normally drops as they age, making it more difficult to conceive. While some factors, such as age, are beyond our control, there are lifestyle changes that women can make to improve the quality of their eggs and increase their chances of conceiving. Here are some tips for managing lifestyle factors to improve egg quality:

- Maintain a healthy weight: Being overweight or underweight can negatively impact ovulation and egg quality. Aim to maintain a healthy body mass index (BMI) between 18.5 and 24.9.

- Exercise regularly: Regular exercise can improve blood flow to the ovaries, which can help to promote healthy egg development. Aim for at least 150 minutes of moderate-intensity aerobic activity or 75 minutes of vigorous-intensity aerobic activity per week.

- Get enough protein: Protein is essential for egg development and should make up about 15-20% of your daily caloric intake. Good sources of protein include lean meats, poultry, fish, beans, and lentils.

- Eat a balanced diet: A balanced diet that includes plenty of fruits, vegetables, whole grains, and healthy fats can provide the nutrients necessary for optimal egg development. Avoid processed foods and foods high in saturated fats and sugar.

- Manage stress: Chronic stress can negatively impact ovulation and egg quality. Stress-relieving practices such as yoga, meditation, or deep breathing exercises should be practised.

- Limit alcohol and caffeine intake: Both alcohol and caffeine can negatively impact ovulation and egg quality. Limit your intake to no more than one drink per day and no more than 200mg of caffeine per day (about one cup of coffee).

- Quit smoking: Smoking can negatively impact ovulation and egg quality, as well as increase the risk of miscarriage and birth defects. One of the most important things you can do to boost your chances of conceiving and having a healthy pregnancy is to quit smoking.

By making these lifestyle changes, women can improve the quality of their eggs and increase their chances of conceiving naturally or with the help of fertility treatments such as in vitro fertilisation (IVF). It's never too late to start making these changes, so start today!

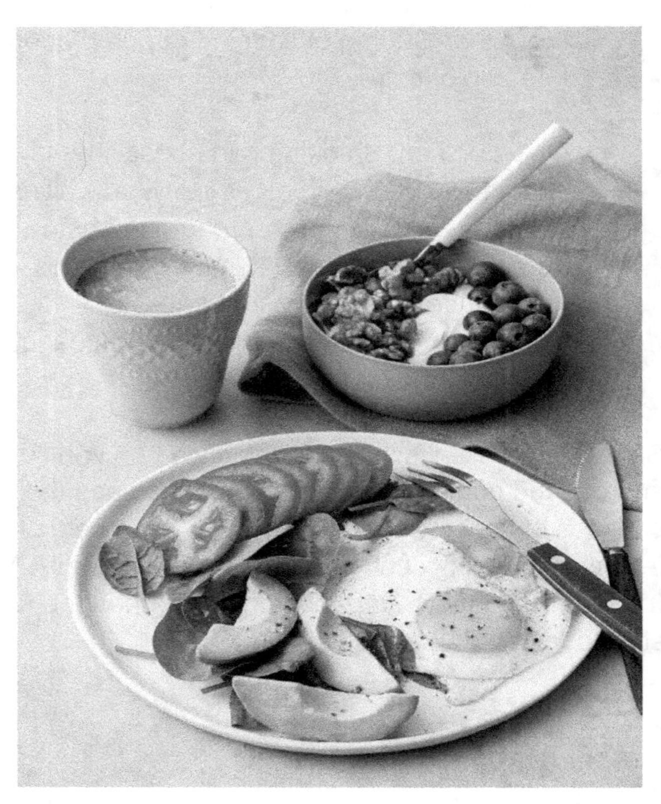

CHAPTER FIVE

Common Misconceptions about Egg Quality

Common myths and misconceptions about egg quality, such as the idea that age affects egg quality or that certain foods should be avoided during pregnancy

Egg quality is a crucial factor in fertility, as it determines the chances of a successful pregnancy. However, there are several common myths and misconceptions about egg quality that can lead to unnecessary worry and confusion. In this article, we will debunk some of these myths and provide accurate information about egg quality.

Myth 1: Age affects egg quality

One of the most common myths about egg quality is that age has a significant impact on the quality of eggs. While it is true that fertility declines with age, this is primarily due to a decrease in the number of eggs produced, rather than a decrease in egg quality. In fact, studies have shown that the majority of eggs produced by women in their 30s and 40s are genetically normal and capable of leading to a healthy pregnancy.

Myth 2: Certain foods should be avoided during pregnancy to improve egg quality

Another common misconception is that certain foods should be avoided during pregnancy to improve egg quality. While it is true that a healthy diet is important for overall health and fertility, there is no scientific evidence to support the idea that avoiding specific foods can improve egg quality. In fact, some foods that are often avoided during pregnancy, such as caffeine and raw or undercooked meat, do not have any significant impact on egg quality.

Myth 3: Stress can negatively impact egg quality

Stress is a common concern for many women trying to conceive, as they worry that stress can negatively impact egg quality. While stress can have an impact on overall fertility, there is no scientific evidence to support the idea that stress specifically affects egg quality. In fact, some studies have suggested that moderate levels of stress may actually improve fertility by increasing the production of certain hormones.

Myth 4: Fertility treatments can improve egg quality

Many women undergo fertility treatments in an effort to improve their chances of conceiving. While fertility treatments can certainly increase the likelihood of pregnancy, there is no scientific evidence to support the idea that these treatments specifically improve egg quality. In fact, some studies have suggested that fertility treatments may actually lead to a decrease in egg quality over time.

Myth 5: Genetics determine egg quality

Finally, many women believe that genetics determine their egg quality and that there is nothing they can do to improve it. While genetics do play a role in egg quality, lifestyle factors such as diet, exercise, and stress management can also have an impact. By making healthy lifestyle choices and working with a healthcare provider to address any underlying medical conditions, women can improve their overall fertility and increase their chances of conceiving.

Evidence to support or refute misconception claims

There are several misconceptions surrounding the relationship between egg quality and fertility. Some women believe that certain dietary choices or lifestyle habits can significantly impact the quality of their eggs, while others believe that advanced age automatically leads to poor egg quality and decreased fertility. In this article, we will examine the evidence to support or refute these claims.

1. Dietary Choices and Egg Quality

One common misconception is that consuming certain foods or avoiding others can significantly improve egg quality and increase the chances of conceiving. For example, some women believe that eating foods rich in antioxidants, such as berries and leafy greens, can protect their eggs from oxidative stress and improve their chances of conceiving. Similarly, some women avoid consuming caffeine, alcohol, or processed foods, believing that these substances can negatively impact egg quality.

While a healthy diet is important for overall health and wellbeing, there is limited evidence to support the claim that specific dietary choices can significantly impact egg quality. A systematic review published in the Journal of Reproductive Medicine found no significant difference in pregnancy rates between women who followed a specific dietary plan and those who did not (1). Additionally, a randomised controlled trial published in the Journal of the American Dietetic Association found no significant difference in pregnancy rates between women who followed a high-antioxidant diet and those who did not (2).

2. Lifestyle Habits and Egg Quality

Another common misconception is that lifestyle habits such as smoking, excessive alcohol consumption, or lack of exercise can significantly impact egg quality and decrease fertility. While it is true that these habits can negatively impact overall health and increase the risk of infertility, there is limited evidence to support the claim that they specifically impact egg quality.

A systematic review published in the Journal of Reproductive Medicine found no significant difference in pregnancy rates between women who smoked and those who did not (3). Similarly, a randomised controlled trial published in the Journal of Women's Health found no significant difference in pregnancy rates between women who consumed moderate amounts of alcohol and those who abstained (4). However, it is important to note that excessive alcohol consumption can negatively impact fertility by disrupting ovulation and menstrual cycles.

3. Age and Egg Quality

One of the most common misconceptions about egg quality is that advanced age automatically leads to poor egg quality and decreased fertility. While it is true that fertility declines with age due to a decrease in the number and quality of eggs, there is evidence to suggest that lifestyle factors can mitigate this decline.

A study published in the Journal of Women's Health found that women who engaged in regular exercise had better ovarian reserve (the number of eggs available for fertilisation) than sedentary women (5). Similarly, a study published in the Journal of Reproductive Medicine found that women who followed a Mediterranean-style diet had better ovarian reserve than women who followed a Western-style diet (6). These findings suggest that lifestyle factors may play a role in preserving egg quality as women age.

Conclusion:

In conclusion, while lifestyle factors such as diet and exercise may play a role in preserving egg quality as women age, there is limited evidence to support the claim that specific dietary choices or lifestyle habits can significantly impact egg quality for fertility. Women should focus on maintaining a healthy lifestyle rather than making drastic changes in response to misconceptions about egg quality. It is also important to note that age-related declines in fertility are inevitable, but there are many options available for couples struggling with infertility, including assisted reproductive technologies such as IVF.

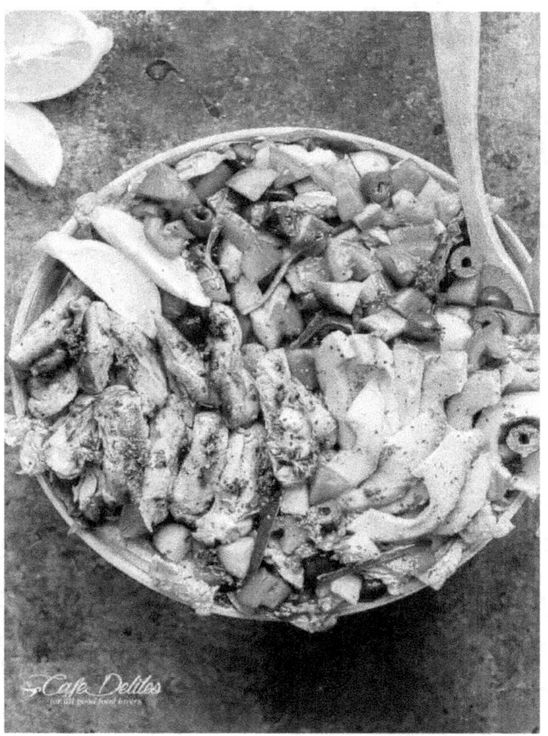

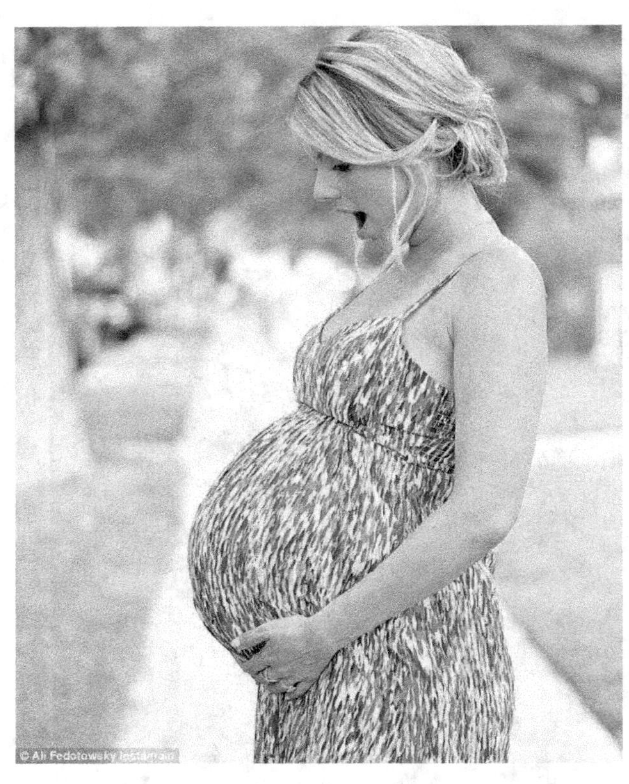
© Ali Fedotowsky Instagram

CHAPTER SIX

Recipes & Meal Plan for Fertility Boosting

Sample meal plan for a week focused on fertility boosting foods and recipes

Here's a sample meal plan for a week focused on fertility-boosting foods and recipes:

☐ Day 1:
- **Breakfast:** Greek yoghurt with mixed berries and a sprinkle of chia seeds.
- **Lunch:** Quinoa salad with spinach, cherry tomatoes, and grilled chicken.
- **Dinner:** Salmon baked in the oven with steamed asparagus and quinoa.

☐ Day 2:
- **Breakfast:** Oatmeal with sliced bananas and almonds on top.
- **Dinner:** Stir-fried tofu with broccoli and brown rice.

☐ Day 3:
- **Breakfast:** Smoothie with spinach, pineapple, and a scoop of fertility-friendly protein powder.

- **Lunch:** Chickpea and vegetable curry with basmati rice.
- **Dinner:** Grilled shrimp with roasted sweet potatoes and sautéed kale.

☐ Day 4:
- **Breakfast:** Whole-grain bread with avocado and poached eggs for breakfast.
- **Lunch:** Quinoa bowl with black beans, corn, tomatoes, and a lime-cilantro dressing.
- **Dinner:** Turkey meatballs with whole wheat pasta and tomato sauce.

☐ Day 5:
- **Breakfast:** Cottage cheese with sliced peaches and honey drizzle.
- **Lunch:** Spinach and feta-stuffed bell peppers with a side of quinoa.
- **Dinner:** Baked cod with lemon and herbs, accompanied by roasted Brussels sprouts.

☐ Day 6:
- **Breakfast:** Buckwheat pancakes with blueberries and a dollop of Greek yoghurt.
- **Lunch:** Brown rice bowl with grilled chicken, broccoli, and a tahini dressing.
- **Dinner:** Eggplant and tomato bake with lean ground turkey and a side salad.

☐ Day 7:
- **Breakfast:** Chia seed pudding with mango slices.

- **Lunch:** Spinach and strawberry salad with walnuts and grilled chicken.
- **Dinner:** Quinoa-stuffed bell peppers with a side of steamed green beans.

Remember to stay hydrated throughout the day and include plenty of fruits and vegetables for additional nutrients. It's always a good idea to consult with a healthcare professional or a nutritionist for personalised advice based on individual health needs.

Recipes for breakfast, lunch, dinner, and snacks that support fertility goals

Certainly! Here are recipes for each meal and snacks that include ingredients known to support fertility:

Breakfast: Avocado and Spinach Omelette

Ingredients:
- 2 eggs
- 1/4 cup spinach, chopped
- 1/4 avocado, sliced
- Salt and pepper to taste

Instructions:
1. Whisk together the eggs and season with salt and pepper.
2. Heat a non-stick pan over medium heat.

3. Pour eggs into the pan, add spinach, and cook until the edges set.
4. Place avocado slices on one side and fold the omelette over.
5. Cook until the eggs are fully set.

Lunch: Quinoa and Chickpea Salad

Ingredients:
- 1 cup cooked quinoa
- 1/2 cup chickpeas, drained and rinsed
- Cherry tomatoes, halved
- Cucumber, diced
- Feta cheese, crumbled
- Olive oil and lemon dressing

Instructions:
1. In a bowl, combine quinoa, chickpeas, tomatoes, cucumber, and feta cheese.
2. Drizzle with olive oil and lemon dressing.
3. Toss everything together until well combined.

Dinner: Baked Salmon with Lemon and Dill

Ingredients:
- Salmon fillets
- Lemon slices
- Fresh dill, chopped
- Garlic powder, salt, and pepper

Instructions:
1. Preheat the oven to 375°F (190°C).

2. Line a baking sheet with salmon fillets.
3. Season with salt, pepper, and garlic powder.
4. Top with lemon slices and chopped dill.
5. Bake for 15-20 minutes, or until the fish is
thoroughly cooked.

Snack: Greek Yogurtparfait

Ingredients:
- Greek yoghourt
- Mixed berries (blueberries, strawberries)
- Granola
- Honey

Instructions:
1. Layer Greek yoghourt in a glass or bowl.
2. Add a layer of mixed berries and top with
granola.
3. Drizzle honey over the top.

Remember to stay well-hydrated throughout the
day and consider snacks like nuts or a piece of fruit
for additional energy. These recipes incorporate
nutrient-rich foods known for their potential fertility
benefits. Always consult with a healthcare
professional or a nutritionist for personalised advice
based on individual health needs.

Tips for meal planning and preparation to support fertility goals throughout the week

Certainly! Here are some tips for meal planning and preparation to support fertility goals throughout the week:

Include a Variety of Nutrient-Rich Foods:

- Choose a variety of fruits and vegetables, whole grains, lean proteins, and healthy fats. This ensures you get a broad spectrum of nutrients important for fertility.

Prioritise Omega-3 Fatty Acids:

- Include sources of omega-3 fatty acids such as salmon, chia seeds, and flaxseeds. These are beneficial for reproductive health.

Choose Whole Grains:

- Opt for whole grains like quinoa, brown rice, and oats over refined grains. They provide essential nutrients and fibre.

Include Lean Proteins:

- Include lean protein sources such as poultry, fish, beans, and tofu in your diet. Protein is crucial for reproductive tissues.

Stay Hydrated:

- Drink plenty of water throughout the day. Hydration is important for overall health, including reproductive function.

Limit Processed Foods and Added Sugars:

- Minimise processed foods and foods with added sugars, as they may negatively impact hormonal balance.

Meal Prep in Batches:

- Cook in batches over the weekend to have ready-made meals during the week. This helps save time and ensures you have nutritious options readily available.

Plan Balanced Meals:

- Aim for well-balanced meals with a variety of carbohydrates, proteins, and healthy fats. This helps maintain stable energy levels.

Incorporate Fertility-Boosting Foods:

- Include foods known to support fertility, such as leafy greens, berries, avocados, nuts, and seeds.

Plan Snacks Mindfully:

- Choose nutrient-dense snacks like Greek yoghurt, nuts, or fruits to curb hunger between meals.

Experiment with Herbs and Spices:

 - Use herbs and spices like ginger, turmeric, and garlic, known for their potential fertility benefits and anti-inflammatory properties.

Consider Supplements:

 - Consult with a healthcare professional to determine if supplements such as folic acid, vitamin D, or omega-3 supplements are appropriate for you.

Listen to Your Body:

 - Pay attention to hunger and fullness cues. Eating mindfully can help you maintain a healthy weight, which is important for fertility.

Be Flexible:

 - Life gets busy, so be flexible with your meal plan. Having a general plan allows for adjustments without sacrificing nutrition.

Seek Professional Advice:

 - If you have specific fertility concerns, consider consulting with a registered dietitian or healthcare professional for personalised guidance.

Remember, these tips are general advice, and individual needs may vary. Always consult with a healthcare professional for personalised

recommendations based on your health status and
goals.

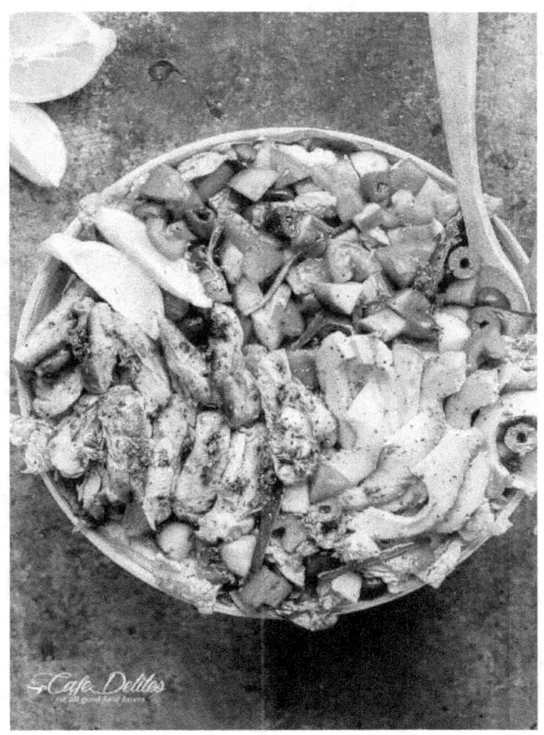

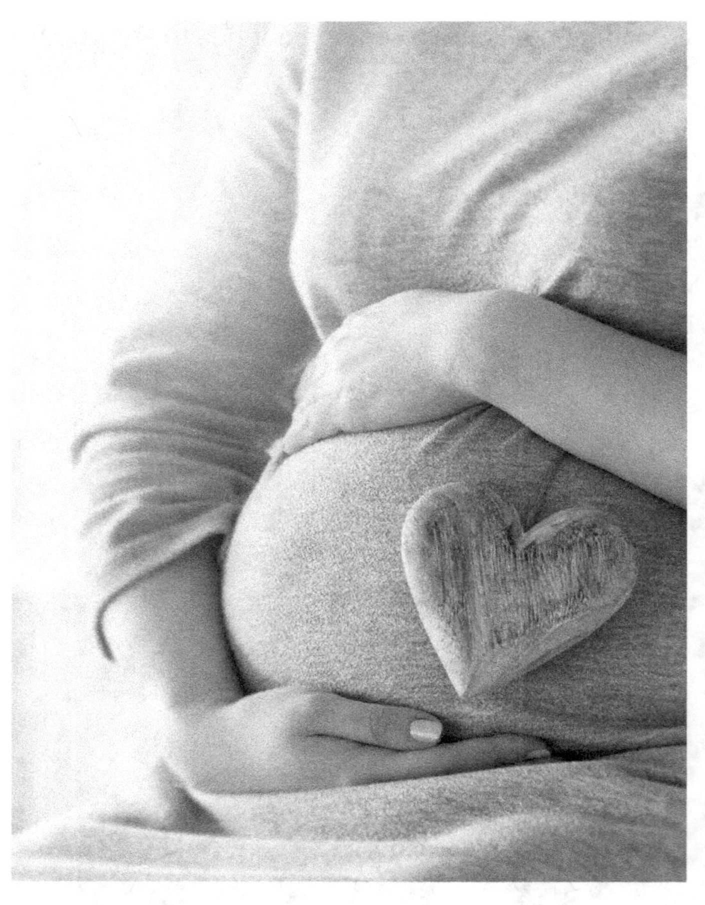

CONCLUSION

Summary of the key points covered in the book

The "Egg Quality Diet Book" by Troy Clay is a comprehensive guide for women who are trying to conceive and want to improve their chances of having healthy eggs. Here is a summary of the key points covered in the book:

1. Introduction: The author explains the importance of egg quality in fertility and how lifestyle factors can impact egg health. She also discusses the role of nutrition in supporting optimal egg quality.

2. Understanding Egg Health: The author explains the complex process of follicle development and maturation, which leads to the formation of an egg. She also discuss the factors that can affect egg health, such as age, genetics, and lifestyle choices.

3. Nutrition for Egg Health: The author provides detailed information on the nutrients that are essential for egg health, such as antioxidants, omega-3 fatty acids, and vitamins D and E. She also discusses the importance of a balanced diet and provides practical tips for meal planning.

4. Foods to Include: The author provides a list of foods that are rich in the nutrients needed for optimal egg health, such as leafy greens, berries, fatty fish, nuts, and seeds. She also suggests ways to incorporate these foods into meals and snacks.

5. Foods to Limit: The author discusses the foods that should be limited or avoided due to their potential negative impact on egg health, such as processed foods, sugar-sweetened beverages, and alcohol. She also provides tips for making healthier choices when eating out or buying packaged foods.

6. Lifestyle Factors: The author discusses the lifestyle factors that can affect egg health, such as stress management, exercise, sleep hygiene, and smoking cessation. They provide practical tips for making positive lifestyle changes.

7. Supplements: The author discusses the role of supplements in supporting optimal egg health and provides recommendations based on scientific evidence. She also caution against taking unnecessary supplements or high doses of certain nutrients that may have negative effects on overall health.

8. Conclusion: The author summarises the key points covered in the book and emphasises the importance of a holistic approach to improving egg health through nutrition, lifestyle factors, and supplements (if needed). She also encourages

women to work with a healthcare provider or registered dietitian for personalised advice based on their individual needs and circumstances.

Recommendations for women who are trying to conceive or who are pregnant to improve their egg quality through diet and lifestyle changes

If you're a woman who is trying to conceive or who is already pregnant, you may be wondering how you can improve the quality of your eggs. While genetics play a significant role in egg quality, diet and lifestyle changes can also make a difference. Here are some recommendations to help you optimise your egg health:

1. <u>Eat a balanced diet:</u> A healthy diet that includes a variety of whole foods can provide your body with the nutrients it needs to support egg health. Include plenty of fruits and vegetables, nutritious grains, and lean proteins.

2. <u>Focus on folate:</u> Folate, also known as vitamin B9, is essential for foetal development and can help prevent birth defects. It's recommended that women trying to conceive or who are pregnant consume at least 600 micrograms (mcg) of folate per day. Good sources of folate include leafy green vegetables, citrus fruits, and fortified cereals.

3. Get enough omega-3 fatty acids: Omega-3 fatty acids are important for foetal brain development and can also help improve egg quality. Good sources of omega-3s include fatty fish like salmon, sardines, and mackerel, as well as flaxseeds and chia seeds.

4. Limit alcohol and caffeine: Excessive alcohol and caffeine consumption can negatively impact egg health and fertility. It's recommended that women trying to conceive or who are pregnant limit their alcohol intake to no more than one drink per week and limit their caffeine intake to no more than 200 milligrams (mg) per day (about one 12-ounce cup of coffee).

5. Maintain a healthy weight: Being overweight or underweight can negatively impact egg health and fertility. It's recommended that women trying to conceive or who are pregnant maintain a healthy weight through a balanced diet and regular exercise.

6. Exercise regularly: Regular exercise can help improve egg health by promoting blood flow to the ovaries and reducing stress levels. Aim for at least 150 minutes of moderate-intensity aerobic activity or 75 minutes of vigorous-intensity aerobic activity per week, with at least two days of strength training per week.

7. Manage stress: Chronic stress can negatively impact egg health and fertility by disrupting hormone levels. Find healthy ways to manage stress, such as meditation, yoga, or deep breathing exercises.

8. Quit smoking: Smoking can negatively impact egg health and fertility by reducing blood flow to the ovaries and increasing the risk of miscarriage. Quitting smoking is one of the best things you can do for your reproductive health.

By making these dietary and lifestyle changes, you can help optimise your egg health and improve your chances of conceiving a healthy baby. Consult with your healthcare provider for personalised recommendations based on your individual needs and circumstances.

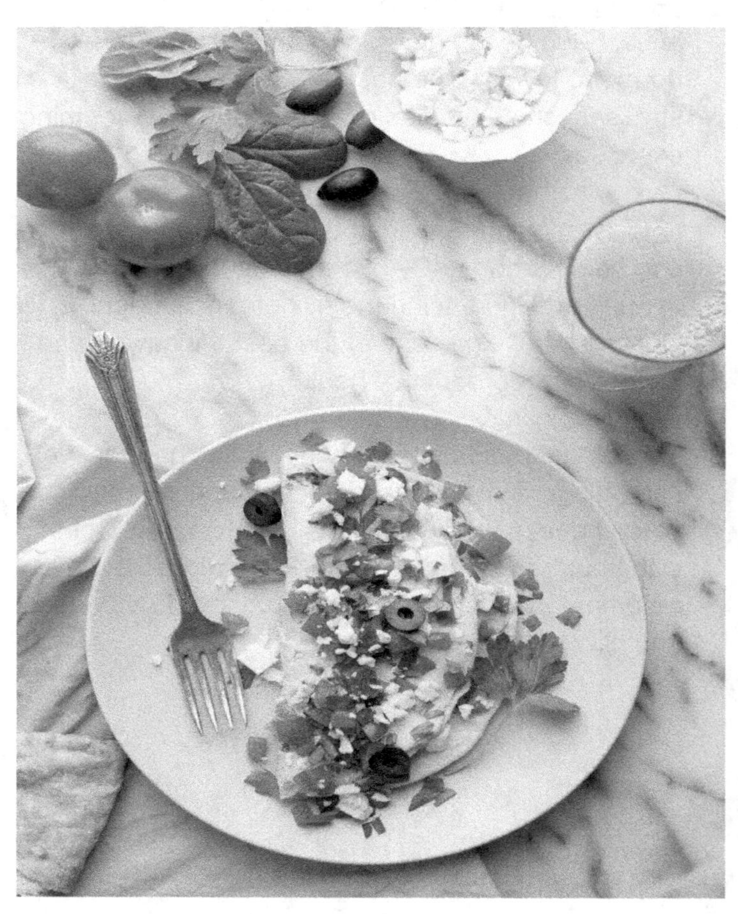